Intermittent Fasting

How to Burn Fat with Intermittent Fasting and Build Muscle, including Sample Meal Plans

Table of Contents

Introduction

Thank you for taking the time to purchasing this book: Intermittent Fasting: How to Burn Fat with Intermittent Fasting and Build Muscle, including Sample Meal Plans

This book covers the various methods of Intermittent Fasting, explains how it works, benefits of fasting, how to incorporate muscle building and provides some same meal plans.

The format of this book allows you to jump right into one of the Intermittent Fasting methods. You can start today. Then you can continue reading to find out more details of how it works.

At the completion of this book you will have a good understanding of Intermittent Fasting and be able to burn fat and build muscle.

Once again, thanks for purchasing this book, I hope you find it to be helpful!

Chapter 1
About Intermittent Fasting

Intermittent Fasting is not a diet fad or a diet plan; rather, it is a way of eating. Intermittent Fasting helps you to determine how to schedule your meals in a way so that you can reap maximum benefit from them. Basically, Intermittent Fasting does not control or change what you eat - it just changes the time of your meals.

But, why is it so important that you change your eating schedule?

Well, it is one of the best ways to lose weight and get a leaner body, without cutting down your calorie consumption or going on a crazy diet plan! As a matter of fact, once you start Intermittent Fasting, you need to keep your calorie consumption the same- you will just eat larger meals in a shorter time span! Also, Intermittent Fasting is a good way to gain muscle mass while losing the excess fat from your body.

One of the main reasons that people opt for Intermittent Fasting is so that they can lose fat – especially the stubborn abdominal fat.

To put it simply, Intermittent Fasting is one of the simplest and easiest weight loss strategies that you can follow, in order to lose the extra fat, while retaining your lean muscles. The reason why Intermittent Fasting is one of the easiest weight loss strategies is that it requires very little behavioral change.

Intermittent Fasting causes very little upheaval in your day-to-day lifestyle, making it easy to follow, but it is also highly effective – meaning, you reap a lot of benefits while putting in minimal effort.

How does intermittent fasting help in losing weight?

To adequately comprehend how Intermittent Fasting helps with weight loss and losing the excess fat in the body, we need to first understand how the body works and what is the base difference between the fasting state and fed state of the body.

When your body is in the fed state, it is usually digesting the food that has been consumed and absorbing the macro and micro-nutrients from the digested food. On average, your body enters the fed state as soon as you start eating and remains in that state for about four to five hours. This is the time that it takes your body to break down and digest the food that you have consumed, and to absorb all the macro and micro-nutrients from that food. When your body is in the fed state, the insulin levels in your body are high, and this makes it really difficult for your body to burn any fat.

After your body has absorbed all of the macro and micro-nutrients from the digested food, your body goes into a state that is commonly referred to as the "post-absorptive state" – a state where your body is not directly or indirectly processing a meal anymore. This state usually lasts for about 9 to 12 hours AFTER you have consumed your last meal. This is when your body enters into the fasting state. While in the fasting state, the insulin levels in the body are low, making it extremely easy for you to burn the extra fat stored in the body. This fat is usually inaccessible for burning in the fed state but is readily available for burning in the fasting state.

But, because the body doesn't enter a fasting state until about 12 hours after the last meal, it is very rare that our body enters or remains in this fat burning stage. This is because by the time our body enters the fasting state we are already hungry or have already consumed the next meal. For example, if you have breakfast at 8am in the morning, your body enters the fasting state by 8 pm. But, by 1 pm – 2 pm you are already hungry for lunch or have already had lunch. With a mid-day meal, your body enters the fasting state post-midnight.

So, with a regular meal plan, you do not have a 12-hour space between two meals, never giving your body the time to enter a faster fat burning cycle!

So, while following an Intermittent Fasting protocol, you provide a 12-hour time gap between two meals, providing your body with adequate time to burn fat. This is one of the main reasons why while practicing Intermittent Fasting you do not need to change your diet much or starve yourself. Even with your regular eating habits, while following Intermittent Fasting, you will lose weight and fat without any extra exercise!

Things to keep in mind

➤ Initially, you may find the "feeding windows" to be a bit too restrictive. In this case, you need to prepare your body for skipping meals. You can do this by pushing your breakfast back by a few hours after you wake up. Start out by pushing your breakfast until almost 4 hours after you wake up, and slowly increase the time span to 8 hours. This will help you to slowly prepare your body to remain hungry for a few hours.

➤ Don't keep thinking about how daunting fasting is. If you keep concentrating or obsessing over how hungry you are or keep counting minutes until you can eat again, you are just going to make the whole process a lot more difficult and torturous for yourself. Instead, go about working as you normally would. This means no wistful glances at your co-worker downing their favorite whipped topping covered frappe from Starbucks. Concentrate and immerse yourself in the work you need to do and the time will just fly. Skipping breakfast is not a very big deal!

➤ Black Coffee is your best friend. It is your fuel that will see you through until it is time for lunch and it helps in curbing your appetite and hunger pangs. But, this absolutely doesn't mean that you drink gallons and gallons of this stuff! The best way to reap maximum benefit from this fuel is to wait until you reach work (about 2 to 3 hours after you wake up) before you consume a mug of black coffee. This ensures that the black coffee has an appetite suppressing effect on the body. It is also advisable that you consume caffeinated beverages only during your fasting period, and completely avoid them during your eating periods. This ensures that your sensitivity to caffeine is maintained.

➢ Drink lots and lots of water. Every time you feel a hunger pang, drink water. Every time you see someone eating something and feel tempted to get yourself some food as well, drink water. Every time you feel like giving up on fasting, drink water. Water not only helps keep you hydrated, it also makes you feel temporarily full and helps keep hunger at bay for some time. Water has zero calories and does not have a negative effect on your body, so you can drink many glasses of it without any worry.

➢ When it is time for you to break your fast, break it by consuming fruit. One of the first signs of hunger is characterized by the depletion of glycogen in the liver. Fruit is a natural source of sugar. So, when you break your fast with some fruit, what you are doing is providing your body with a quick and easy fix for its problems, immediately reducing the hunger pangs that you may be feeling. In this way, you can further extend your fast by another few hours by only consuming 100 to 170 calories! This will make it easier for you to continue fasting and will also limit the number of calories that you consume.

➢ When you finally start eating, do not stick to a set of rules or instructions. Rather, listen to what your body is communicating to you. You do not want to remain hungry while you are supposed to be eating; this will only end up backfiring terribly in the future. So, if your body says it wants more food, but you've already exhausted the number of calories you can eat in a day, do not remain hungry. Try eating a low calorie, high satiating food item. Some raw, fibrous vegetables are very low in calories and can really help you to feel full. On the other hand, if you feel full even before you reach the number of calories that you need to consume, do not continue eating just for the sake of eating. Listen to your body and stop eating. Overeating is just going to make you feel uncomfortable.

➢ Eat foods that not only fill your caloric requirements but fill your stomach too. You do not want to consume a handful of nuts that help you meet your caloric requirements, but don't do anything to satiate your hunger. Consume a hearty meal that contains a lot of potatoes, fibrous veggies, meat, dark chocolate and some nuts too. Remember, just filling your caloric requirements won't really satisfy your hunger; and if you go to bed hungry you will feel cranky the next day. This kind of a mood will be detrimental to a day of fasting and the urge to cheat or give up will be a lot higher. So, make sure you fill your stomach during your feeding periods!

You do not need to compulsorily consume the usual 3 meals a day or even 2 meals a day. You can consume one large meal and consume a number of small healthy snacks during the feeding period. You are the master of your diet and you can consume whatever you want, whenever you want, during the feeding period. Do not feel like you are constricted to follow certain rules just because everybody follows them. If you feel like eating just before you go to bed, eat a meal before you go to bed- it will NOT affect your fat loss significantly. As long as you are refraining from consuming food for a set number of hours, it doesn't really matter how you consume your calories during your feeding period. So, do not keep stressing about eating three to four proper meals. Intermittent Fasting works best when you listen to your body and go with the flow.

Chapter 2
Most Popular Methods of Intermittent Fasting

Intermittent Fasting has slowly gained popularity in recent years. It has been observed that while following an Intermittent Fasting protocol, one can lose weight, notice a marked improvement in their metabolic health, and even extend longevity in some cases.

With its rising popularity, various Intermittent Fasting methods have been designed, each with their own set of rules. All of these methods work, but their level of effectiveness is highly dependent upon each individual. As each individual's metabolism is different, the methods also have different impacts on each individual. What works best for your best friend may not work for you at all. So, it is advisable that you try a method on a trial basis for a few days before ascertaining whether it works for you or not. Also, please consult your physician before you embark on any of the mentioned methods, especially if you suffer from any diseases, such as Type 2 diabetes, heart problems, Alzheimer's or cancer.

In this chapter, the 6 most popular and highly effective methods will be explained in detail:

The 16:8 Method

The basic concept of the 16:8 method is to fast for about 14 to 16 hours a day and to have a feeding window that lasts about 8 to 10 hours. Within this feeding window, you can fit in about 3 to 4 meals or even smaller meals.

This method is also often referred to as the Leangains method, and Martin Berkhan, a world-renowned fitness expert, made this method popular.

The 16:8 method of fasting is as easy as having an early dinner, no munching after dinner, and then skipping breakfast the next morning.

For example, if you finish your dinner by 9 pm, then don't eat anything until about 1 in the afternoon on the next day. By this strategy, your body remains in the fasting state for a good 4 hours (taking into consideration the fact that your body gets into the fasting state about 12 hours after your last meal.) During these 4 hours of fasting your body is in a constant fat burning cycle that helps you lose weight.

It is usually recommended that women do not fast for more than 14 hours, as their bodies work better during a shorter fasting time frame, rather than a longer one.

The 16:8 method is usually easy to follow, but the people who usually have a heavy breakfast may find it a little unsettling to go hungry in the morning. But, with time, your body easily adjusts to this change in eating habits, and you can ignore the hunger pangs quite easily. On the other hand, regular breakfast skippers find it easy to follow this diet plan, and have been following this diet plan without knowing about it!

One of the things that you can do to reduce your hunger is to consume non-caloric beverages during your fasting periods. This includes water, tea, and coffee. The consumption of these liquids makes your stomach feel heavy, deluding your body into thinking it has eaten something, and reducing the hunger pangs that you may experience.

While there is not really any restriction on the foods that you should eat and the foods that you should avoid consuming during your feeding window, it is advisable that you consume healthy foods, such as salad or baked chicken, as opposed to unhealthy foods, such as deep-fried foods or foods that have a lot of preservatives in them. Remember, the more calories and junk food you eat, the more time your body takes to process the food, thus, reducing your "fasting state".

It is advisable that you eat healthy, nourishing and nutrient rich foods that satiate your appetite, without being too heavy on the stomach. One such diet plan that you can combine with Intermittent Fasting is a low carb diet plan. By going low carb, you restrict your appetite and even reduce it, reducing the urge to eat something during your fasting period. Another advantage of going low carb is that your body shifts to a fat burning state of ketosis, resulting in double the fat loss with minimum effort on your end!

So, remember, skip breakfast and consume your lunch snack/ dinner during the span of 8 to 10 hours and you will be good to go!

The 5:2 Method

The basic premise of the 5:2 diet is to eat normally for 5 days a week while limiting your calories to about 500 calories to 600 calories for the remaining 2 days a week.

This diet was initially popularized by Michael Mosley, a British doctor and journalist, and is also commonly referred to as the "Fast Diet".

It is advised that men should consume no more than 600 calories on the fasting days, while women should limit their calorie intake to about 500 calories during the fasting days. For example, you can eat normally on all days of the week, except on Saturdays and Wednesdays, where you need to eat only two small meals (about 300 calories each for men and 250 calories each for women.

During the 5 non-fasting days of this method, you do not need to count your calories or restrict them in any manner, but it would do well if you consume healthy and nutrition rich foods and avoid all the high-calorie junk foods, to make it easier for your body to adjust to the low-calorie days and to also lose weight effectively.

Initially, you may find it a little difficult to adjust to the restricted calories. You can counter this by scheduling your fasting on days that you are not expected to do a lot of work. In this way, you can prepare your body to survive on minimal calories without stressing it out or feeling weak.

The Eat–Stop–Eat Method

Popularized by Brad Pilon, a fitness expert, the Eat–Stop–Eat method calls for a fast that lasts for 24 hours and should be done twice a week. This can be modified to one fasting day per week if needed. This is one of the most popular methods of Intermittent Fasting.

You can fast from dinner on day one to dinner on day two, successfully fasting for 24 hours. For example, if you complete your dinner on Sunday at about 8 pm, and do not eat anything until Monday 8 pm, you have successfully completed a 24 hour fast.

It is not necessary to fast from dinner to dinner; you can also fast from lunch one day to lunch the next day or even breakfast on one day to breakfast the next day. The meal may change, but the end result remains the same.

During your 24 hours fast, you can consume any beverage that doesn't have calories, such as water, tea or coffee, but you strictly cannot consume any sort of solid food.

If you wish to lose weight by following the Eat–Stop–Eat method, it is extremely important that you consume adequate amounts of calories during your feeding periods. Eat normally; just avoid junk food and heavily processed food, and you should be good to go.

The only problem with this method is the requirement to stay hungry for a full 24 hours. A lot of people may find this method very difficult to follow. It is advisable that you start out slowly. One might do this with fasting periods of about 14 to 16 hours and then slowly increase the fasting period as you feel comfortable.

Initially, you might face ravenous hunger around the 20 to 22 hour mark, but be strong and you will make it through. If you cannot, and you break your fast around the 20 hour mark or the 22 hour mark, do not beat yourself up about it. It happens to the best of us. Take your experience as a lesson and set your mind to complete your fast the next time around.

The Alternate Day Fasting Method

The name "alternate day fasting" is fairly self-explanatory as to what this method entails. To the oblivious, this method involves fasting on every other day, while consuming regular meals on the days you do not fast.

There are various versions of this method. Some methods call for consumption of no food on fasting days, while other methods allow you to consume up to 500 calories on fasting days.

If you are following the no food for 24 hours method, you can suppress your hunger pangs by consuming non-caloric beverages, such as water, tea or coffee. Apart from these beverages, you can consume absolutely no solid food.

If you are following the restricted calories method, you need to restrict your calories to 500 calories on fasting days. These calories can be consumed in a single large meal, say lunch or dinner or over a span of multiple small meals, spread throughout the day.

The various studies that have been conducted to evaluate the benefits of Intermittent Fasting have based their tests on some versions of this particular method of Intermittent Fasting.

A full day of fasting every other day may sound extreme, and it is not advisable that beginners follow the alternate fasting method. This method is not very pleasant to follow. You may end up going hungry a few times a week and the hunger pangs can get a bit annoying after a while. This method is best to follow for a short term; perhaps a week or two, before you revert to another, more sustainable method of fasting.

The Warrior Diet Method

Popularized by Ori Hofmekler, a fitness expert, the Warrior Diet method involves fasting throughout the day while consuming a huge meal at night. Fasting through the day, you are allowed to consume small amounts of raw vegetables and fruits.

Basically, you fast for about 20 hours during the day while giving yourself a small 4-hour feeding window in order to meet your caloric needs.

This method of Intermittent Fasting comes with a set diet plan and it was one of the first diet plans that included Intermittent Fasting in its model. The Warrior Diet plan calls for the consumption of foods that are very similar to the regular Paleo foods – unprocessed foods, whole foods, foods as close to their raw counterparts, etc.

The Warrior Diet aims to mimic the diet of ancient warriors who consumed very little food during the day while consuming whatever they hunted at night. It is called "under-eating" during the day and "over-eating" during the night.

Initially, it will be difficult to switch from a regular meal cycle to a one meal a day cycle, and the sudden shift may lead to you feeling weak or light-headed. You need to gently ease into the rhythm of this diet. You can start out by skipping breakfast a couple of times a week and then slowly increase the number of days, until you skip breakfast every day. Once you have adjusted to skipping breakfast every day, you can then start your lunch skipping cycle until you are well adjusted. It is a slow, frustrating process that requires a lot of patience.

Unlike other fasting methods, you do not need to starve yourself during the fasting period by restricting your consumption to non-caloric beverages such as water, tea or coffee. You can consume raw vegetables or fruits, and even a small amount of protein if you wish. You can even consume freshly pressed juices, but do not consume any canned or processed products.

The portion of protein should not be more than 6 ounces. Some of the proteins that you can consume are yogurt, eggs, poultry, sashimi, etc. One strict guideline you need to follow is that you absolutely should not mix multiple proteins.

The basic rule of eating during the fasting or "under eating" period is that you should feel hungry, but you shouldn't feel the pain of starvation.

While consuming your one meal at night there is no particular time when you need to consume the meal nor any set number of calories that you need to eat. You can eat whatever you want, whenever you want (even right before sleeping!). Eat whatever quantities that you want; the only catch is that you should stick to whole, unprocessed foods and highly saturated foods. It is said that you should eat until you start feeling thirsty, and once you are thirsty you should stop eating!

The Spontaneous Meal Skipping Method

This method calls for the skipping of meals whenever you feel like skipping one. You do not have to follow a fixed structure fasting plan in order to reap the benefits of Intermittent Fasting.

You can skip a meal whenever you are not hungry or do not have the time to cook or just don't feel like eating.

It is a commonly propagated myth that if you do not eat every few hours your body will start losing muscle or your body will go into a "starvation mode". Rather, to the contrary, the human body is built to withstand long periods without food without affecting its regular functioning. So, a few skipped meals here and there aren't really going to have a negative impact on you!

So, if you wake up late and are in a hurry, skip breakfast and eat a wholesome lunch followed by a healthy dinner a few hours later.

Or if you are out and about and cannot find anything that suits your tastes, skip lunch entirely and opt for a healthy dinner a few hours later.

Skipping out on a meal or two when you do not feel like eating or when you want to skip one is known as spontaneous Intermittent Fasting. Just make sure that the meals that you do consume are healthy, nutritious and wholesome. You do not need to compensate for the calories of the skipped meals in the meals that you do consume, so just eat enough to satisfy yourself; do not overeat.

There you have it – the six most popular methods of Intermittent Fasting. Before opting for any of these methods, it is advisable that you consult your dietitian or physician so that you are sure that you are not harming your body in any way.

Chapter 3

Effects of Intermittent Fasting on Metabolism, Hormones, Insulin, and Cells.

When you fast, you will observe changes in your body. But, what you may not know is that the changes that take place in your body are not just limited to what you can observe on the outside. Changes happen on the inside too, on a molecular and cellular level.

For example, once you start Intermittent Fasting, the hormone levels in your body change so that the fat stored in the body is readily accessible for burning. Another change that can be observed in the body is that the cells in your body go into repair mode and this also results in the changes of the expression of genes.

Here is a list of changes that you can expect your body to undergo when you begin an Intermittent Fasting protocol.

Metabolism

A lot of people believe in the myth that when you skip a meal or two you are just slowing down your metabolic rate. According to the myths, this happens because your body wants to save energy for the more important tasks and it starts storing all the extra nutrition for future use.

Well, these myths have got one thing right, that this metabolic slowing does tend to happen. But, what this oversimplified explanation misses out on is that this only happens when you starve your body for very long periods of times. Your body won't go into starvation mode just because you skipped a meal.

However, it has been proven that when you fast for shorter time periods, your metabolism doesn't slow down! Rather, fasting will result in a significant increase in the rate of metabolism.

A study conducted by the Department of Internal Medicine at the University of Vienna in Austria found that when 11 healthy men were made to fast for 3 days. The result was that their metabolism increased by a massive 14%! This increase was due to the increase in the fat burning hormones in the body that are increased due to fasting!

Hormones

Hormones are the messengers in the body. They are the chemical compounds that travel through your body in order to promote growth and metabolism.

Hormones also play a major role in weight regulation in the body. This is due to the impact they have on the amount of food that you eat, your appetite, and the fat that is burned or stored in your body. Intermittent Fasting has been proven to bring about a balance in the fat burning hormones in the body, making it an extremely helpful tool to lose weight.

Human Growth Hormone

Intermittent Fasting promotes the increase in the level of human growth hormone in the blood. This human growth hormone plays an important role in promoting fat loss in the body.

Many studies have shown that the levels of human growth hormone in men can increase by nearly five times while they are fasting!

When there is an increase in the level of human growth hormone in the body, there is not only an increase of fat burning in the body, but there is also a marked increase in the preservation of the body's muscle mass.

Women, on the other hand, do not always reap similar benefits from fasting; at least not at the level that men do. Studies have observed that while there is an increase in human growth hormone in women, the increase is not on par with the levels that men achieve.

Norepinephrine

Norepinephrine is a stress hormone in the body. This hormone is responsible for your attention and alertness to your surroundings. Norepinephrine also contributes to the split-second response that your body has to external and internal stimuli.

One of Norepinephrine's other functions is to cause the fat cells in the body to release their internal fatty acid so that they can be easily broken down.

So, when there is an increase of the norepinephrine hormone in the bloodstream, there is a larger amount of fat available for your body to break down and burn.

While fasting, your body experiences a lack of ready sources of energy to burn. This causes your body to release more norepinephrine into the bloodstream, in order to release more fatty acids. This process further results in the breakdown of fat to provide your body with much-needed energy.

Insulin

Insulin is one of the most important hormones to be associated with the fat burning metabolism of the body. The presence of insulin signals to your body that there is enough glucose to fuel the body and the body should store the fat from the meals and not burn it.

With high levels of insulin present in the body, losing weight becomes an extremely difficult task. High levels of insulin can also result in, or be a result of, various diseases, such as Type 2 diabetes, cancer, cardiovascular diseases and obesity.

Intermittent Fasting helps in the reduction of insulin levels in the body; something very similar to the impact that low carb diets have on the body.

When you restrict your intake of carbohydrate-rich foods, the body runs out of glucose to produce energy. Your body then shifts to a fat burning metabolic state known as ketosis.

Intermittent Fasting may not put your body into a state of ketosis, but it brings it close enough for your body to start burning fat. When burning fat becomes the body's primary fuel source, the body's insulin levels automatically decreases.

It has been observed that Intermittent Fasting can bring down the insulin levels in the body by a whopping 20% -30%!

Cells

Does fasting help in making the cells in our body more damage resistant? Are the benefits just temporary during the time of fasting, or are they long lasting? A group of scientists decided to find out, and here is what they discovered:

Anti-Aging Benefits

Over the years, scientists have been trying to find the health benefits that one can reap by limiting the number of calories one consumes.

One of the most prominent theories suggests that the health benefits from limiting caloric intake are primarily due to the decrease in blood sugar levels in the body. When the level of blood sugar is low, our cells are forced to work more in order to provide the body with an alternative source of energy.

A study conducted using Rhesus monkeys has shown that when the monkeys are only provided about 70% of the calories that they normally consume, they tend to live a longer and healthier life. And this phenomenon is not just limited to the Rhesus monkeys. Many other animals were subjected to Intermittent Fasting. They consumed the regular quantity of calories for a day and restricted calories for the next day and similar results were observed. Recently, studies conducted on humans have shown similar effects of anti-aging.

But, why does fasting have such an impact on our body?

Repairing the cells damaged by free radicals

One of the most common ways by which our cells get damaged is oxidative stress. When you prevent the cells from getting damaged due to oxidative stress, or repair the damaged cells, your body doesn't age as much as it regularly would.

But why does oxidative stress occur? It occurs when there is a large production of free radicals in the body. These unstable molecules carry a bunch of highly reactive electrons.

When these free radicals come across another molecule, they try to combine with it, by either giving up an electron to the molecule or taking in an electron from the molecule. In both cases, a chain reaction follows. This results in the formation of more free radicals that go on to break apart more and more molecules.

Some of the molecules destroyed can be important components of essential proteins, cells, DNA or cell membranes. The presence of antioxidants in the body ensures that there are enough "free molecules" in the body to combine with these free radicals so that the important cells and other important parts of the body do not get damaged.

Free radicals can develop in the body when the mitochondria do not function optimally. When you switch to intermittent fasting, you reduce the glucose levels in the body, forcing your body to switch to other "difficult" sources of energy, such as burning of fatty acids. When your body makes this switch, it forces the cells to expel the faulty mitochondria and replace them with healthy and properly functioning mitochondria. This results in the lowered production of free radicals in the body.

And this is how Intermittent Fasting has a long-lasting impact on the body, by bringing about a change at the cellular level, promoting better growth and reducing the aging of the body.

Chapter 4
How Intermittent Fasting Burns Fat

We all have read about how Intermittent Fasting promotes fat burning in the body, but in this chapter, it will be explained exactly how Intermittent Fasting can help the body to become a fat burning machine.

Your body is forced to burn belly fat while intermittent fasting

When you consume a meal, the blood sugar levels in your body rise. The sugar present in the blood is then used, along with the glycogen and carbs already stored in the body, to produce energy for the day to day functioning of the body and for the performance of various tasks.

When you first begin fasting, you do not consume a meal for a couple of hours. When this happens, your blood sugar level decreases. Your body starts burning its stored carbohydrates and glycogen to provide your body with enough energy to perform its normal functions.

Once your body runs out of the stored carbs, your body has no option but to start burning its stored fat. The body will start metabolizing fat in order to perform its normal bodily functions, as well as to provide you with enough energy to perform various tasks.

The fat present in your body is just a buildup of all the times you overate or all of the extra calories left behind when you did not perform enough physical functions to burn them.

When there are extra calories left over in your body, the body does not simply excrete them; these calories are meticulously saved by the body for future use. They will be used when you do not consume enough food to provide your body with energy or when you exercise more and do not eat enough.

So, when there is not enough blood sugar in the body to see you through, the body starts burning its leftover fats to keep itself going. So, the fewer carbs you consume, the less blood sugar in the body. The less blood sugar in the body, the more fat you burn!

Your metabolism increases during intermittent fasting

Your blood sugar levels dramatically decrease when you start fasting. Your body's response to this lowered amount of blood sugar is to provide you with more energy by releasing norepinephrine into the bloodstream.

As explained before, norepinephrine is a stress hormone. It not only helps in making you feel more alert and focused, but it also helps you to start burning the extra fat in the body. This provides your body with much-needed energy.

Belly fat loss is one of the main targets of intermittent fasting

Abdominal fat is stubborn. It is more difficult to shed abdominal fat than any other bodily fat stores. This is because your abdominal area contains a larger amount of alpha–2 receptors. These receptors slow down the fat-burning process in the body, while the beta–2 receptors increase the fat burning process in the body.

With the level of insulin going down in the body, the amount of alpha–2 receptors decrease, resulting in the activation of the high-fat burning beta–2 receptors in the abdominal region. This helps in burning the highly stubborn belly fat present in the body.

While Intermittent Fasting, there is also a marked increase of blood flow to the belly area, this makes it easier for norepinephrine, the fat burning hormone, to enter the abdominal area and aid in fat burning.

Intermittent Fasting helps in the reduction of stubborn fat in the abdominal, hip, butt and thigh areas. These are the areas where most women have the largest amount of fat built up. This makes Intermittent Fasting especially important for women to follow.

But, you will only start losing belly fat after you lose fat from all over your body. This is because belly fat is stubborn and difficult to breakdown. Fat in other areas is easy to break down and hence, is broken down first.

Once you get into the fat burning rhythm, you will lose all the extra fat in no time at all!

Increase in the level of human growth hormone

As explained before, human growth hormone helps in burning fat, and aids in building and maintaining muscle mass in the body. Studies have shown that Intermittent Fasting increases the levels of human growth hormone by about 2000% in a male's body and by about 1300% in a female's body.

Human growth hormone is also responsible for maintaining muscle mass while you fast. According to a study conducted by the Department of Kinesiology and Nutrition at the University of Illinois, it is proven that while following Intermittent Fasting, there is better maintenance of muscle mass as opposed to other diets and fads.

If you are still not convinced, look through videos of Hugh Jackman, who followed Intermittent Fasting in order to build muscle mass and lose fat, in order to prepare his body to play Wolverine!

Intermittent fasting helps in reducing your appetite

It is a simple principle: the lesser amounts of food that you eat, the faster you will lose weight!

When you begin an Intermittent Fasting protocol, you may experience extreme hunger pangs and cravings. But as your body adapts to the change in your meal cycle, and as you mentally accept the change, you will find that the food cravings become less severe. This is because Intermittent Fasting helps in the balancing of ghrelin. Ghrelin is a hormone responsible for hunger, so balancing it results in a reduced appetite.

While you are practicing Intermittent Fasting, you will probably consume only 1, 2 or at the most, 3 meals in a day, depending on which method you follow. Once your body is adapted to your Intermittent Fasting protocol, you will feel limited hunger. But, when you consume your normal meal cycle of 3 to 6 meals a day, you will feel hungrier and your appetite will increase considerably.

The bottom line is that Intermittent Fasting helps in losing fat faster because:

1. Your hunger and cravings reduce significantly, leading to a lower appetite and consumption of food.

2. Due to the reduced levels of insulin in the body, and the increased levels of human growth hormone, you will burn more calories and fat. Most of which is already stored in your body.

Chapter 5

How to Incorporate Building Muscle During Intermittent Fasting

In recent years, many people have become curious about Intermittent Fasting. There may be a variety of reasons for this increasing interest. These reasons range from wanting to lose fat the easy way, to peoples' busy lifestyles. Many have no inclination to cook multiple meals a day. Some people also have busy schedules where they are unable to squeeze in a lunch or a breakfast.

In some cases, Intermittent Fasting is followed by people due to certain beliefs. For example, by Muslims when they fast during Ramadan or otherwise from about 5 am to 7 pm.

Whatever your reasons may be, you may have wondered how you can build up any muscle mass while following this eating schedule. A lot of people assume that it is next to impossible to gain muscle mass while fasting. The fact is that if you spend a little time to plan out your day and your meals in the correct way, you can easily build muscles while fasting!

Here are some of the things that you should keep in mind in order to maximize your success.

Opt for training sessions that are scheduled late at night

If you are fasting for a specific time period where you will be fasting from a set time in the morning to a set time in the evening (for example the Ramadan fasting set up of 5 am to 7 pm), it is best if you place your workout sessions for after 7 pm, as waking up and working out before 5 am will be a Herculean task.

It is always advisable that you consume some food before you start with your resistance-training program, so doing your training session before 7 pm is extremely unlikely. You also need to consume a certain amount of carbohydrates and proteins after your training program is over so that your body can begin the recovery process. You will not be able to do this if you are supposed to be fasting for that particular time period.

When you start with a late evening training session, you can make sure that you consume your dinner immediately once you are home from work or as soon as your fasting period ends. This meal can act as a "pre-fuel" before you begin working out.

You can then start your training session, once you are done eating, say at around 7:30 pm and continue training for an hour or however long your workout lasts, giving you time to finish it by say 9 pm. This will give you enough time to squeeze a post workout meal into your schedule until it is time for bed at around 10 pm.

Consume the bulk of your caloric requirement after your training session

The second most important thing for you to do while following this protocol is to be sure that you consume the bulk of your required caloric intake immediately after you finish working out. As mentioned before, this post workout meal helps the body with regeneration. By helping the body to recover from the workout, this post workout meal aids in the generation of lean muscle mass in the body.

For this to work, you first need to figure out the number of calories that you need to consume in a day so that you can build up adequate amount of muscle mass. Once you figure out your total caloric needs for the day, consume about 20% of the required calories right before you begin working out. This meal should contain both carbohydrates and proteins, as this meal will act as a fuel for your workout. If you do not consume adequate carbs or proteins, you will feel extremely lethargic and tired.

After you finish your daily workout, the post workout meal should consist of about 60% of your total required calories. These calories can also be divided into 2 or 3 small meals in the time span that ranges from post work out to bedtime.

This meal is likely to contain a large number of calories that you need to consume in a short span of time. You may find it difficult to consume the required quantity of calories all together. It helps to focus on consuming foods that have a large number of calories, such as red meat, dried fruit, bagels, raw oats, etc.

You should also keep in mind that the meal you are consuming is immediately after you finish working out. So, with this kind of a meal plan set up, you should consume high carb foods that will help in building muscle, rather than opting for foods that are high fat and low carb. This is because immediately after working out, your body requires carbohydrates. In this scenario, if you provide your body with more fat, it will have a detrimental effect on your body.

This doesn't mean that you have to eliminate all the fat from your diet. You can consume a meal that has a lot of carbs or proteins just after you finish your training and then consume a high fat or high protein meal just before you sleep. The point is to keep the fat consumption low in the meal that immediately follows the workout session.

Fatty foods are more calorie-dense and it is extremely easy to eat them in a large amount, for example, nuts, butter, oils, etc. These are easier to consume than a lot of high carb foods – especially when you are already feeling satiated. So, it is best if fatty foods are consumed as a second small meal just before bed, while carbs are consumed immediately after working out.

Try to squeeze in a meal before 5 am

The last thing that you need to do while following this approach to building muscle while Intermittent Fasting is to eat a meal immediately after you wake up. For all of the people who aren't following Ramadan and are just fasting to lose weight/gain muscle mass, this meal can be consumed at whatever time you naturally wake up.

If you are following Ramadan, it is advisable that you wake up earlier, say around 4:30 am, just before the fast begins, and consume a slow digesting protein, such as red meat with some cottage cheese, that will make up for the remaining 20% calories that you need to consume.

You can also add in some fat or carbs to this meal, but make sure that you consume about 35% of your required protein at this time. This ensures that there is a steady supply of amino acids in the body while you fast throughout the day.

After consuming the meal, you can go back to sleep if you want.

Make sure that when you follow this type of muscle building Intermittent Fasting regimen, that you keep all of the aforementioned points in mind. If you try to perform a large volume of highly intense exercise while consuming very few calories, your body will react negatively to it and you will do yourself more harm than good.

Slowly, the body will lose all the stored glycogen and will be deprived of it. This will result in lethargy, the inability to keep up with your workouts and the incapability to recover. To be sure that this doesn't happen to you, you will need to force feed yourself until your body becomes acclimated to this meal cycle. Eventually this approach will start feeling normal to you and your body.

Chapter 6
Benefits of Intermittent Fasting

Intermittent Fasting is not a regular diet that dictates what you should eat and what you should avoid eating. Rather, Intermittent Fasting is a meal schedule plan that consists of alternate periods of feeding and fasting.

Since the dawn of time, the ancient human has followed Intermittent Fasting – directly or indirectly. The cave man hunted during the day and due to his inability to carry a lot of supplies, he ate little or nothing during the day and satisfied his hunger with one meal at night. Intermittent Fasting is based on this cycle of fasting and feasting.

Over time, the popularity of Intermittent Fasting has increased, leading to a number of studies being conducted in order to measure the benefits that one can reap by following Intermittent Fasting – benefits that affect the body as well as the mind.

This chapter contains a list of 10 benefits of Intermittent Fasting, backed with evidence, which shows how good this way of life really is!

Positive impact on the hormones, cells and genes

When you do not consume food for a certain time period, there are many changes that take place in your body. For example, as explained in a previous chapter, your body initiates a crucial damaged mitochondrial replacement that has an anti-aging effect on the body. Another very important change is that there is a marked increase in the release of various hormones in the body. These hormones aid in the fat burning process in the body.

Here is a list of few changes that you can expect to occur in your body once you begin an Intermittent Fasting protocol:

➢ The insulin levels in the body drop, which makes the process of fat burning a lot easier. This is because when you restrict your food consumption, you are reducing the levels of blood glucose. In order to keep the body running, the body then shifts to a fat burning metabolic cycle, resulting in the reduction of fat storage in the body.

➢ The level of human growth hormone in the blood stream increases by almost fivefold in the body while practicing Intermittent Fasting. This elevated level of human growth hormone in the blood helps with the burning of fat in the body, and aids in building lean muscle mass.

➢ When the glucose levels in the body drop, your body is forced to look for an alternative source of energy. This alternative source of energy is usually the excess fat that is stored in the body. As fats are more difficult to breakdown than the usual glucose molecules, your cells are forced to work harder and more efficiently. One of the effects of this is that in order to work more efficiently, the cells repair the dysfunctional mitochondria. It is these broken mitochondria that are responsible for producing free radicals in the body, leading to the slow oxidation of cells, DNA, cell membranes, etc. So, when these mitochondria are replaced, your body slowly ensures that you age at a slower rate!

➤ The replacement of mitochondria doesn't just affect the life of the cells, but also has an impact on the genes. These genes do not get oxidized, and live longer, thus leading to better protection against various diseases.

➤ Intermittent Fasting also leads to the release of norepinephrine in the body. This is not just responsible for keeping you alert, focused and for regulating your "fight or flight" response. It is also responsible for initiating the breakdown of the stored fats into fatty acids, further leading to quick fat loss.

Loss of excess weight and abdominal fat

Let us face the fact that you probably heard of Intermittent Fasting when you started researching about the best and most efficient way to lose weight and fat. The basic idea of Intermittent Fasting is to consume fewer meals. So, unless you are trying to consume enough calories in order to make up for the calories missed out during skipped meals, you will end up consuming a lot fewer calories than you would have normally consumed.

Intermittent Fasting, as explained before, has an impact on the fat burning hormones in the body, leading to an increased production of human growth hormone and norepinephrine in the body. These two hormones not only perform their assigned roles, but they also help in initiating the fat burning action in the body.

Combine the increased hormones with low levels of insulin in the body and you will find that there is a marked increase in the breakdown of the stored fat in the body to be used to provide the body with some much-needed energy.

It is due to this very reason that short term fasting leads to an increase in the metabolic rate of the body by about 4% to 15%. This means that your body burns calories even while you are at rest!

So, to put it simply, Intermittent Fasting helps you in both ways; the increased metabolic rate helps with the burning of the calories in the body, while there is also marked reduction in the amount of food and calories you consume.

According to a report published by the Department of Kinesiology and Nutrition, University of Illinois, Chicago, back in 2014, it was observed that Intermittent Fasting could lead to a weight loss of about 3% to 8% over a span of 3 to 24 weeks. This is a huge amount of weight loss for the little work you are required to put in!

It was also observed that the people who took part in the study lost a lot of inches from their waistlines, ranging from about 4% to 7%. This is a clear indication that they not only lost weight but also lost a lot of the stubborn abdominal fat. This fat is usually the cause for a lot of diseases!

Another study, also conducted by the Department of Kinesiology and Nutrition, at The University of Illinois, has shown that while there is some muscle loss while Intermittent Fasting, this muscle loss is a lot less when compared to other diets and fads; especially restricted calorie consumption over a period of time.

Lowering the risk of Type 2 diabetes

Type 2 diabetes has become increasingly common in the past few decades, with the number of people affected by the disease increasing almost fourfold between 1980 and 2014. One of the main features of Type 2 diabetes is abnormally high blood sugar levels due to the development of insulin resistance in the body.

Insulin resistance is when the muscles, liver cells, and fat in the body do not respond to the insulin in the bloodstream and are unable to absorb the glucose from the blood. In order to counter this, the body prepares higher levels of insulin so that these body parts respond to the insulin and absorb the required glucose. As long as the beta cells in the body can keep up with this increased insulin demand, the body functions normally. But, once the beta cells start lagging, there is marked increase in the glucose levels in the blood, resulting in various health issues, one of them is diabetes.

So, anything that helps in the reduction of insulin resistance in the body indirectly helps in the lowering of the blood sugar levels, further protecting the body against Type 2 diabetes.

Intermittent Fasting has shown to reduce the insulin resistance in the body, which also leads to a massive reduction of the blood glucose levels. In the studies that have been conducted, it was observed that fasting insulin levels were reduced by almost 20% to 30% and fasting blood sugar levels had been decreased by about 3% to 6%.

Another study conducted by the Laboratory of Chromatin Biology, Department of Pharmacology and Toxicology, at the

National Institute of Pharmaceutical Education and Research, Punjab India, on diabetic rats showed that Intermittent Fasting not only reduced the insulin and blood sugar levels in the rats but also helped in preventing kidney damage – a severe complication that is suffered by a lot of diabetes patients.

This shows that Intermittent Fasting may have a protective effect on people who are at a high risk of contracting Type 2 diabetes.

However, the impact of Intermittent Fasting on diabetes patients is volatile and there is a varied effect on different genders. For example, a study conducted at the Pennington Biomedical Research Center, in Baton Rouge, Louisiana, revealed that the blood sugar control actually took a turn for the worse while following a 22-day long Intermittent Fasting cycle.

So, if you suffer from Type 2 diabetes or are pre-diabetic it is advisable that you consult your dietitian or local physician before embarking upon the Intermittent Fasting journey.

Reduction of inflammation and oxidative stress in the body

Oxidative stress is one of the main reasons that our body ages and we slowly head towards a number of chronic diseases. As explained earlier, oxidative stress is when free radicals in the body (produced due to faulty mitochondria in the cells of the body) react with the molecules in the body and break them apart. These free radicals are unstable molecules and they react with various important molecules, such as cells, genes, cellular membranes,

DNA, etc. and either take an electron from those molecules or give them an electron, making them unstable.

Several studies have shown that by following Intermittent Fasting, you can decrease the oxidative stress in the body and increase your body's resistance to it. This is because when you practice Intermittent Fasting, you reduce your body's reliance on glucose as a source of energy and force your body to shift to a fat burning cycle. This shift requires the cells to work harder. In order to keep up with this increased load, cells concentrate on making themselves more efficient by expelling the damaged and faulty mitochondria. This lowers the number of free radicals floating around in the body and also reduces the oxidative stress in the body.

Other studies have also shown that Intermittent Fasting can help counter inflammation. Inflammation is another major reason why the body faces a number of common and chronic diseases.

Good for the Heart

Heart disease is one of the largest causes of death around the world today, with it being the cause for 1 out of 4 deaths in the US. This is extremely alarming since most of the risk factors responsible for causing heart disease are linked to your weight; such as high blood sugar, high cholesterol, high blood pressure, obesity, sedentary lifestyle, etc.

It would appear that the obesity epidemic that we are seeing today is having a rather disastrous impact on our lives.

Intermittent Fasting helps in improving a number of the aforementioned risk factors. Firstly, it helps you shed the extra weight and extra fat from your body; and as we all know, obesity is the root cause for most of the risk factors mentioned earlier.

Secondly, Intermittent Fasting helps in reducing the "bad" cholesterol levels in the body. LDL is the bad cholesterol and smaller particles of LDL wreak more havoc in your body than larger particles. While Intermittent Fasting, the LDL count in the body is reduced by about 25% and there is a remarkable decrease in the smaller particles too. There is also a marked decrease in the triglycerides in the body by about 32%. Triglycerides are a kind of fat cell that are used to store the extra energy from the meals that you consume. High levels of triglycerides in the body can lead to insulin resistance and instances of acquiring cardiovascular disease.

According to a study conducted on 19 healthy volunteers, it was observed that when they were subjected to 24-hours of fasting, followed by a fixed calorie meal, there was a marked decrease in the inflammation in the body while fasting.

Another study conducted by Department of Surgery, Louisiana State University Medical Center, in New Orleans, Louisiana, has shown that when adults suffering from asthma were subjected to an alternate day fasting meal plan, there was a striking decrease in the regular oxidative stress markers, inflammation, and other symptoms in the body!

Cell repair processes

When you practice an Intermittent Fasting regimen, the glucose levels in your body go down. In order to keep your body up and running, your body starts breaking down the stored fat in the body as an alternative source of energy.

Now, the reason glucose is the primary source of energy for our body is that glucose is one of the easiest molecules to break down. As compared to glucose, fat is a lot more complicated to break down and our cells need to work a lot harder to extract energy from it.

In order to remain efficient, cells begin repairing the damaged cells and remove all the waste. This process is known as autophagy. This process involves the gradual breakdown of cells followed by the metabolism of all the dysfunctional and broken proteins that tend to accumulate inside the cells over a period of time.

This increased autophagy helps to provide the body protection against a number of diseases, such as Alzheimer's disease and cancer.

Possible protection against cancer

Cancer is one of the worst diseases on this planet and is usually characterized by the unrestrained and out of control growth of cells in the body. Intermittent Fasting has been observed to have several benefits, including a few effects on the metabolic cycle of the body that increase the body's resistance to cancer.

Although most of the studies have been conducted on lab animals, the success of these tests would make one believe that indeed there is something worth looking at with a human perspective.

Another study conducted by the Andrus Gerontology Center and Department of Biological Sciences, at the University of Southern California, in Los Angeles, has shown that fasting by cancer patients helped them by reducing the various side-effects one may feel while undergoing chemotherapy.

Good for brain health

As a general rule of thumb, whatever is good for the body is also good for the brain. Intermittent Fasting acts upon various metabolic functions that are known to be factors which help in improving the health of the brain.

This is because Intermittent Fasting promotes good cell growth and helps in reducing the oxidative stress in the body. It also reduces the inflammation that happens in the body. Intermittent Fasting also helps in bringing down the blood sugar levels and reducing insulin resistance.

Several studies, conducted on lab animals, have shown that Intermittent Fasting also helps in promoting the growth of new and improved nerve cells in the body, providing the body with a higher level of brain function.

Intermittent Fasting is also known to increase brain-derived neurotrophic factor, the brain hormone, in the body. The deficiency of this brain hormone is often implied to be the cause of various brain-related problems, including depression.

Animal studies also suggest that Intermittent Fasting can effectively help safeguard the brain against strokes.

May help in the prevention of Alzheimer's disease

Alzheimer's disease is a type of dementia and is considered to be a neurodegenerative disease. It is one of the most common types of dementia across the world.

Alzheimer's has absolutely no cure. It is extremely important to safeguard yourself against this disease and to prevent it from happening to you!

A study conducted on rats has shown that Intermittent Fasting helps in delaying the onset of Alzheimer's in certain cases while reducing its severity in other cases.

In a couple of case reports presented by the Mary S. Easton Center for Alzheimer's Disease Research, Department of Neurology, University of California, Los Angeles, and The Buck Institute for Research on Aging, it was observed that a change in lifestyle that included short-term fasts on a daily basis had a significant impact on abating and improving the symptoms of Alzheimer's in 90% of the patients observed.

Animal studies conducted at Sanders-Brown Research Center on Aging and Department of Anatomy and Neurobiology, University of Kentucky, in Lexington, have suggested that Intermittent Fasting can also help in protecting the body against a number of neurodegenerative diseases that include Huntington's disease and Parkinson's disease.

Extends your lifespan

One of the most interesting effects of Intermittent Fasting is the effect it has on your lifespan and the ability to extend it.

According to the research conducted at Department of Psychosomatic Medicine, Graduate School of Medical Sciences, Kyushu University, in Fukuoka, Japan on lab rats, it was observed that there was a dramatic increase in the lifespan of the rats. In some of the studies, it was seen that rats who were subjected to alternate day fasting lived a considerably longer life than the rats that were fed on a daily basis. To be precise, fasting rats lived for a whopping 83% longer.

Intermittent Fasting, as explained before, reduces the oxidative stress on the body due to its effects on cellular repair. This reduced oxidative stress is caused by the reduction of the free radicals in the body that are responsible for increased molecular damage to cells, cell membranes, DNA, genes, etc. Once this molecular damage is reduced, it has an anti-aging effect on the body, as your body repairs and replaces damaged cells constantly.

As it is evident from this chapter, Intermittent Fasting has a great impact on the body. All you need to do is time your meals properly and you should see some great benefits!

Chapter 7
Sample Meal Plans

Intermittent fasting is not a diet plan that dictates what you should eat and what you should avoid eating. Intermittent fasting provides you with a schedule of when you need to consume a meal and at what time.

Meal plans vary from method to method, from person to person, as no two physiques are the same, nor will two bodies react to foods in the same manner. In this case, it is important to understand your dietary and caloric needs and plan your meals according to them.

16:8 Method

If you are following the Leangains method of intermittent fasting that uses a 16:8 ratio of fasting to feeding time period, your schedule should look as follows:

Time / Day	Sun	Mon	Tue	Wed	Thu	Fri	Sat
Midnight to 4am	Sleep/ Fast	Sleep/ Fast	Sleep/ Fast	Sleep/ Fast	Sleep/ Fast	Sleep/ Fast	Sleep/ Fast
4am to 8am	Sleep/ Fast	Sleep/ Fast	Sleep/ Fast	Sleep/ Fast	Sleep/ Fast	Sleep/ Fast	Sleep/ Fast
8am to Noon	Fast	Fast	Fast	Fast	Fast	Fast	Fast
Noon to 4pm	Eat	Eat	Eat	Eat	Eat	Eat	Eat
4pm to 8pm	Eat	Eat	Eat	Eat	Eat	Eat	Eat
8pm to Midnight	Fast	Fast	Fast	Fast	Fast	Fast	Fast

Your meal consumption during these days is highly dependent upon the number of calories that you need to consume in a day. The number of calories that you are required to consume depends on your current weight, goal weight, level of activity, etc.

24 Hour Fasting

One of the quickest and best ways to begin intermittent fasting is to begin slowly by squeezing in a 24 hour fast once a week. It helps in preparing your body for fasting, and provides your body with most of the health benefits of fasting without having to cut down on the number of calories you consume.

As you can see in the table below, you need to stay hungry for 24 hours, once a week. This 24-hour time period can be any time, from dinner on day one to dinner on day two, lunch on day one to lunch on day two or breakfast on day one to breakfast on day two.

Time / Day	Sun	Mon	Tue	Wed	Thu	Fri	Sat
Midnight to 4am	Sleep/ Fast	Sleep/ Fast	Sleep/ Fast	Sleep/ Fast	Sleep/ Fast	Sleep/ Fast	Sleep/ Fast
4am to 8am	Sleep/ Fast	Sleep/ Fast	Sleep/ Fast	Sleep/ Fast	Sleep/ Fast	Sleep/ Fast	Sleep/ Fast
8am to Noon	Eat	Fast	Fast	Eat	Eat	Eat	Eat
Noon to 4pm	Eat	Eat	Fast	Eat	Eat	Eat	Eat
4pm to 8pm	Eat	Fast	Eat	Eat	Eat	Eat	Eat
8pm to Midnight	Eat	Fast	Eat	Eat	Eat	Eat	Eat

Alternate Day Intermittent Fasting

Alternate day intermittent fasting calls for longer fasting periods at regular intervals through the week. For example, as evident from the table below, you would eat dinner on Monday and then fast until you eat dinner on Tuesday. On Wednesday, you eat the whole day, but avoiding eating anything on Thursday until dinnertime. This allows your body to effectively follow long fasting period, while providing you with a minimum of one meal a day, even on fasting days!

Time / Day	Sun	Mon	Tue	Wed	Thu	Fri	Sat
Midnight to 4am	Sleep/ Fast	Sleep/ Fast	Sleep/ Fast	Sleep/ Fast	Sleep/ Fast	Sleep/ Fast	Sleep/ Fast
4am to 8am	Sleep/ Fast	Sleep/ Fast	Sleep/ Fast	Sleep/ Fast	Sleep/ Fast	Sleep/ Fast	Sleep/ Fast
8am to Noon	Eat	Eat	Fast	Eat	Fast	Eat	Fast
Noon to 4pm	Eat	Eat	Fast	Eat	Fast	Eat	Fast
4pm to 8pm	Eat	Eat	Fast	Eat	Fast	Eat	Fast
8pm to Midnight	Eat	Fast	Eat	Fast	Eat	Fast	Eat

Sample Meal Plan

Here is a sample meal plan for a person who weighs about 220 pounds. There are two meal plans, one for the day when they work out for at least an hour, while another for the rest of the days.

Workout day

Meal #1: To be consumed between noon to 1 pm

1. 3.5 ounces oats

2. 4 large egg whites

3. 0.3 ounces Sunflower, flax, pumpkin and sesame seeds

4. 3 caps of 6 Omega

5. 1 Scoop of Whey Protein

6. 0.3 ounces almonds

7. 0.17 ounces of 100% cacao (nibs or powder)

Total calories consumed: 739

Meal #2: To be consumed between 4 pm to 5 pm

1. 5.2 ounces brown rice

2. 5.2 ounces chicken breast, fat removed

3. 4.7 ounces green beans

4. 0.6 ounces almonds

5. 1 medium tomato and 1 medium bell pepper

6. 4 large egg whites

Total calories consumed: 634

Meal #3 + Meal #4: To be consumed between 8 pm to 9pm

1. 5.2 ounces brown rice

2. 5.2 ounces chicken breast, fat removed

3. 4.7 ounces green beans

4. A shake made using 1.4 ounces glucose powder and 2 scoops of whey

5. 1 medium tomato and 1 medium bell pepper

6. 1.4 ounces almonds

7. 6 large egg whites

8. 1 large egg yolk

Total calories consumed: 1255

Total calories consumed in the day: 2625

Rest Day

Meal #1+ Meal #2: To be consumed between noon and 1 pm

1. 11 ounces oats

2. 10 large egg whites

3. 0.3 ounces Sunflower, flax, pumpkin and sesame seeds

4. 3 caps of 6 Omega

5. 1 Scoop of Whey Protein

6. 1.4 ounces almonds

7. 0.17 ounces of 100% cacao (nibs or powder)

8. Shake made using 2 scoops of Whey

Total calories consumed: 1113

Meal #3: To be consumed between 4 pm and 5 pm

1. 1.7 ounces brown rice

2. 5.2 ounces chicken breast, fat removed

3. 4.7 ounces green beans

4. 1 medium tomato and 1 medium bell pepper

5. 3 large egg whites

6. 1 large egg yolk

7. 0.7 ounces almonds

Total calories consumed: 578

Meal #4: To be consumed between 8 pm and 9 pm

1. 1.7 ounces brown rice

2. 5.2 ounces chicken breast, fat removed

3. 4.7 ounces green beans

4. 1 medium tomato and 1 medium bell pepper

5. 3 large egg whites

6. 1 large egg yolk

7. 0.7 ounces almonds

Total calories consumed: 578

Total calories consumed in the day: 2247

Now, this diet plan should only be followed if you are going to exercise a minimum of one hour on workout days with a more than sedentary level of exercise on rest days (30 minutes of brisk walking or 15 minutes of jogging). This meal plan should effectively explain to you how you need to break down your required calories over the span of 8 to 9 hours, and the amount of food that you should consume in a day.

This sample meal plan contains a moderate to large amount of carbohydrates and proteins and a low amount of fats. This is because carbs and proteins are required in order to help the body recuperate after working out and also help in building lean muscles mass.

You can tweak the quantities of the macronutrients according to your needs.

Conclusion

Thanks again for taking the time to purchasing this book!

You should now have a good understanding of Intermittent Fasting, and be able to burn fat and build muscle.

If you enjoyed this book, please take the time to leave me a review on Amazon. I appreciate your honest feedback. It greatly helps me to continue producing high quality books.

www.ingramcontent.com/pod-product-compliance
Lightning Source LLC
Chambersburg PA
CBHW071118280526
45787CB00003B/1086